SPECIAL OPERATIONS FITNESS

by
Life is a Special Operation.com

SPECIAL OPERATIONS FITNESS

Copyright © 2017 by Littlestone

All rights reserved. No part of this publication may be reproduced, distributed or transmitted in any form or by any means, without prior written permission.

Special Operations Fitness / Paperback -- 1st ed.
ISBN: 978-1-946373-06-9
$34.99 everywhere great books are sold

Special Operations Fitness / E-book -- 1st ed.
ISBN: 978-1-946373-07-6
$24.99 at www.lifeisaspecialoperation.com

LIFE IS A SPECIAL OPERATION.COM

Table of Contents

About Special Operations Fitness 5
Special Operations Fitness Training Philosophy 6
- ★ Train as you Fight: 6
- ★ Individual Discipline and Motivation: 6
- ★ Short Duration Workouts: 6
- ★ Don't Over-Train: 6
- ★ Self Defense: 7
- ★ Proper Running Technique: 7
- ★ Save your Knees and Joints: 7
- ★ Crosstrain: 7
- ★ You Don't need Expensive Gear or Equipment: 7
- ★ Discipline is Essential 7
- ★ Diet is Essential: 8
- ★ Sleep is Essential: 8
- ★ Plan Ahead: 8
- ★ Dress Appropriately: 8
- ★ Timing: 8
- ★ Warm Up Before. Only Stretch After: 9
- ★ Long, Fast Walks: 9
- ★ Safety: 10

Special Operations Fitness 11
Special Operations Fitness Work Outs 12
- Fitness Test 12
- United States 13
- Canada 14
- Mexico 15
- Guatemala 16

SPECIAL OPERATIONS FITNESS

Belize 16

El Salvador 17

Honduras 18

Nicaragua 18

Costa Rica 19

Panama 20

Self Defense 1 21

Self Defense 2 21

Self Defense 3 22

Self Defense 4 22

Self Defense 5 22

Self Defense 6 23

Bike 1 "Tour De Neighborhood" 24

Bike 2 "Seatless in Seattle" 25

Swim 1 "Tsunami" 25

Swim 2 "Flash Flood" 26

"1000 Week" 27

Cross Train 1 & 2 27

2 or 3 Hour Walks 27

4, 5, 6 or 7 Hour Walks 28

5 Essential Training Tips to Prepare for Special Forces or Delta Force Selection 28

The 6th Essential Training Tips to Prepare for Ranger School 30

Special Operations Fitness Exercises 31

Special Operations Fitness Self Defense Techniques 32

Conclusion 32

Progress Tracker 34

LIFE IS A SPECIAL OPERATION.COM

ABOUT SPECIAL OPERATIONS FITNESS

Greetings, my name is Christopher Littlestone and I am the creator of Special Operations Fitness. My obsession with fitness began three decades ago when I was a Junior in the Arizona public school system. I had just been selected to be the Cross Country Team Captain, yet was the slowest runner on the team. It was then that I realized that I was more gifted with "leadership" than with elite physical strength and agility. Ever since then, I have had to trained harder and smarter than all my colleagues so that I could maintain the world-class physical fitness and endurance levels required to survive rigorous Special Operations training and missions.

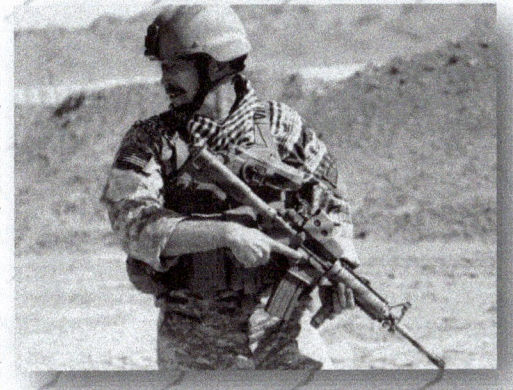

My credentials… I am a retired U.S. Army Special Forces (Green Beret) Lieutenant Colonel who has been an elite athlete for over 30 years. I have a Master's Degree from Harvard and am a Special Forces Combat Diver, an Airborne Ranger, and a decorated war veteran who has spent over 10 years serving outside of the United States.

Our Team… The Special Operations Fitness team consists of elite soldiers and police, an engineer, a pharmacist, a few random geniuses, the camera crew and a web designer… only real people doing real fitness.

During my 3rd Deployment to Afghanistan

The average week consists of 4 workouts, three during the week and one on the weekend. The week day workouts are high intensity but short duration. The weekend workout is a variation of cross training or a long hike.

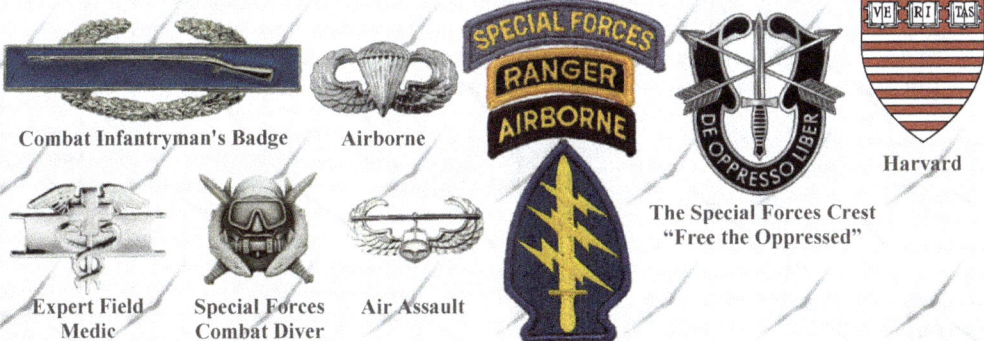

Combat Infantryman's Badge | Airborne | The Special Forces Crest "Free the Oppressed" | Harvard
Expert Field Medic | Special Forces Combat Diver | Air Assault

SPECIAL OPERATIONS FITNESS

SPECIAL OPERATIONS FITNESS TRAINING PHILOSOPHY

Special Operations Fitness believes that "Life is a Special Operation." We want to enjoy life and get the most out of life. Being smart, healthy and physically fit makes you feel better and makes life much easier. Our basic principles are listed below:

★ <u>Train as you Fight:</u> Special Operations Fitness is going to help you build muscle, strength, health, and confidence so you are fully prepared for the challenges of your life. Hopefully you will never be in a fight. But you are likely to face a crisis or potential challenge. A crisis is usually a short sprint, not a long run. This is why we will emphasize high intensity explosive exercises. Running away from an out-of-control car requires sprinting. Fighting off a potential rapist requires explosive power and energy. Because we want you to "train as you fight," we ask that you give us 100% for every workout.

> **SPECIAL OPERATION FITNESS** is a 12-week unconventional training program designed to shred body fat, increase cardio vascular efficiency and muscular strength, teach or reinforce essential self-defense techniques, build confidence, and increase physical and mental performance.

★ <u>Individual Discipline and Motivation:</u> Without individual discipline, there is no way to be the best of the best. Inspiration and motivation must come from within. Although working in a team is always a good way to keep you accountable, you are not competing with or against a team. You are competing against yourself in an attempt to be stronger, smarter, and more physically fit than you have ever been. All workouts are individual. But feel free to working out with a "Fitness Buddy" or in a small group.

★ <u>Short Duration Workouts:</u> A short duration, high intensity workout is the best way to make get ripped, keep your cardio vascular system working at maximum efficiency, and build and keep muscle.

★ <u>Don't Over-Train:</u> Many athletes train 7 days a week. This is too much. The body never gets to rest and recover. Furthermore, Special Operations Forces exist to conduct Special Operations, not train. Training is only preparation for the Operation. Since "Life is a

Special Operations," we don't want to waste our entire lives training, we want to spend most of our time enjoying.

★ Self Defense: Special Operations Fitness includes 10 Self Defense sessions. These Self Defense workouts focus on basic boxing and kicking techniques and are guaranteed to "wear you out." Whether an experienced warrior or an amateur soccer mom, you will benefit from these challenging and confidence building workouts.

★ Proper Running Technique: Using proper running technique increases speed and cardio vascular efficiency, reduces muscular-skeletal impact, and decreases the probability of injury. We wish every kid had to take track and field "sprinting" workshops in school. Once you learned how to run properly, you instantly feel and see the difference. It is never too late to learn proper form: Don't heal strike. Land on your mid or forefoot. Swing your arms front and back, not sideways. Head up. Knees high. Torso erect, slightly forward leaning. Fast cadence. Use your hamstrings… Please learn how to run properly. Your joints will thank you.

★ Save your Knees and Joints: Most exercise programs out there place undue stress on your knees and joints. Doing 100 swinging pullups is a great way to injure yourself. Running every day is going to blow out your knees. Special Operations Fitness believes that short, intense workouts are better for your joints than long ones. We believe in sprinting, rather than jogging.

★ Crosstrain: By mixing up and changing your workouts, your body will always be challenged, adapting, and growing stronger. Special Operations Fitness provides dozens of work outs and exercise variations guaranteed to turn your body into an elite and efficient machine.

★ You Don't need Expensive Gear or Equipment: Special Operations Fitness minimizes the use of equipment. We require that you have a punching bag (Heavy Bag), hand wraps, punching bag gloves, a Pull Up bar, a Low Pull Up bar, and a couple of Dumbbells. You can buy these tools for life long use, use equipment at a gym or a friend's house, or make some of them yourself. Be flexible and adapt.

★ Discipline is Essential: Discipline and unwavering resolve are always required to be the best of the best. Thousands of people waste money paying Personal Trainers each week to hold their hand from fitness machine to machine, even though they already know how the machine works. This is because they lack discipline. Please "Ranger Up" and find, make, or build the discipline required to finish this life changing Special Operations Fitness program.

SPECIAL OPERATIONS FITNESS

★ <u>Diet is Essential:</u> To be a world class performer you need to be fueled by real (not processed) food. No one puts cheap gas into a race car. When I was a young Special Forces Officer I lived off of cheeseburgers, protein shakes, and Starbuck's Frappuccino's. I survived, but in spite of my bad eating habits. Once I learned more about the importance of eating healthy, and started to actually eat an abundance of real, healthy food, my performance increased significantly. At Ranger school, students endure a war like environment and are starved of food and sleep. As a result, students are always miserable and their technical performance is not optimal. In contrast, students at the amazingly difficult Special Forces SCUBA School are allowed to eat as much as they want, to include having a midnight snack in their barracks room. The course was still exceptionally challenging, but students were fueled for success. Please feed your body with healthy and real food while conducting the Special Operations Fitness Program. Use the Scuba school nutrition model, not the Ranger school nutrition model.

★ <u>Sleep is Essential:</u> Most people are sleep deprived and functioning below their potential. In order for the Special Operations Fitness program to be a success, you must get eight hours of sleep or more a night. This will help your body to rest and recover, allowing you to physically and mentally perform at optimal levels.

★ <u>Plan Ahead:</u> World class training requires an efficient use of time. For example, every hour of every day of Ranger School is planned for Ranger students and printed on the master training plan (of course the students don't get to see the plan). Special Operations Fitness has made a very detailed fitness plan for you to execute and we recommend that you take a few minutes each week to plan your workouts and routes ahead of time. Plan what and when to eat. Plan when to sleep and when to wake up. Plan where to go to have the required dumbbells and how to get access to a required Heavy Bag during "Self Defense" workout days. Be deliberate and plan ahead so you can successfully complete each workout.

★ <u>Dress Appropriately:</u> We recommend wearing the appropriate, protective clothing when exercising. Usually this means boots, pants and gloves. Swim in pants and a t-shirt. Psychologists have realized that when a person puts on a uniform they become the part. So wear a Special Operations Fitness uniform and you will become more intense, more focused, and it will make things more fun. "Mandex" (Man Spandex) and "Wandex" (Woman Spandex) are unauthorized.

★ <u>Timing:</u> Special Operations Fitness recommends doing the three week-day workouts early in the morning, before work or school. Working out in the morning kick starts your metabolism and gets you energized and burning fat all day long.

LIFE IS A SPECIAL OPERATION.COM

★ Warm Up Before. Only Stretch After: It is important to get your heart pumping and muscles warmed up before starting your workout. A few minutes of biking, jogging, or jumping jacks should do the trick. Never stretch a cold muscle. Stretching a cold muscle is an easy way to tear or injure that muscle. Only stretch after your muscles are warm, but preferably after the workout as part of your cool down. Please warm up before every workout and only stretch after the work out.

★ Long, Fast Walks: Special Forces soldiers and Infantry Men might walk all day. Literally, they might have their backpacks on for 24 hours. Don't forget that an M4 rifle weighs seven pounds or that a M240B machine gun weighs 27 pounds. Not only is long distance walking a significant part of Special Operations training, it can be a low impact exercise beneficial for people of all ages. When you do a long, fast walk you burn calories. But even after you finish a long, fast walk you continue to burn calories. This is why you can go on a backpacking trip, eat chocolate bars all day, and come back skinnier and leaner than when you left. Carrying a heavy backpack and body armor is part of Special Operations, one which frequently causes life-long disabilities in the neck and back. For this reason, we don't recommend heavy backpacks during walk days. Beginners can carry food and water and safety gear but experts should not exceed 30 pounds. The added physical stress of carrying a weapon will be simulated by carrying a small 3-5 pound dumbbell. You will shred away calories, burn fat, build core body muscles, get fresh air, and enjoy hours of low impact, high benefit walking.

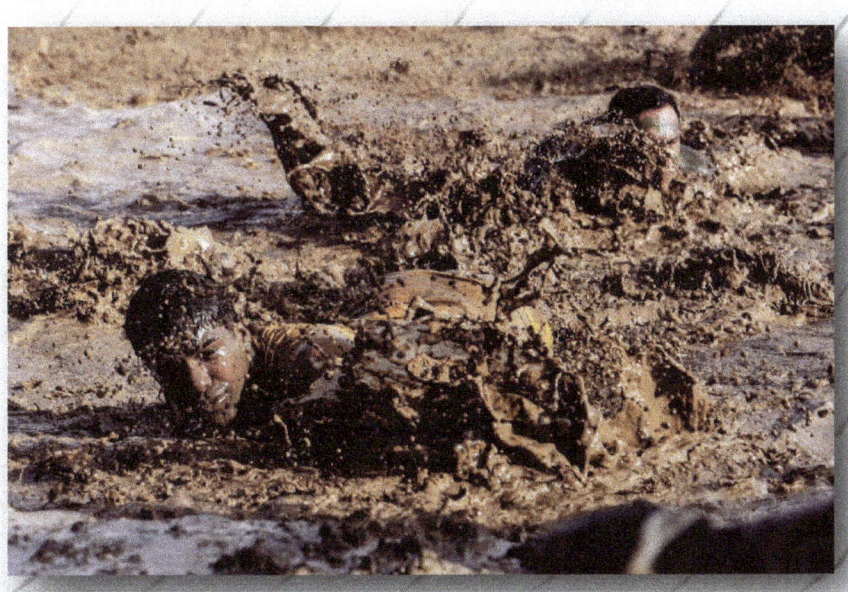

Muddy Obstacle Course... Dress Appropriately

SPECIAL OPERATIONS FITNESS

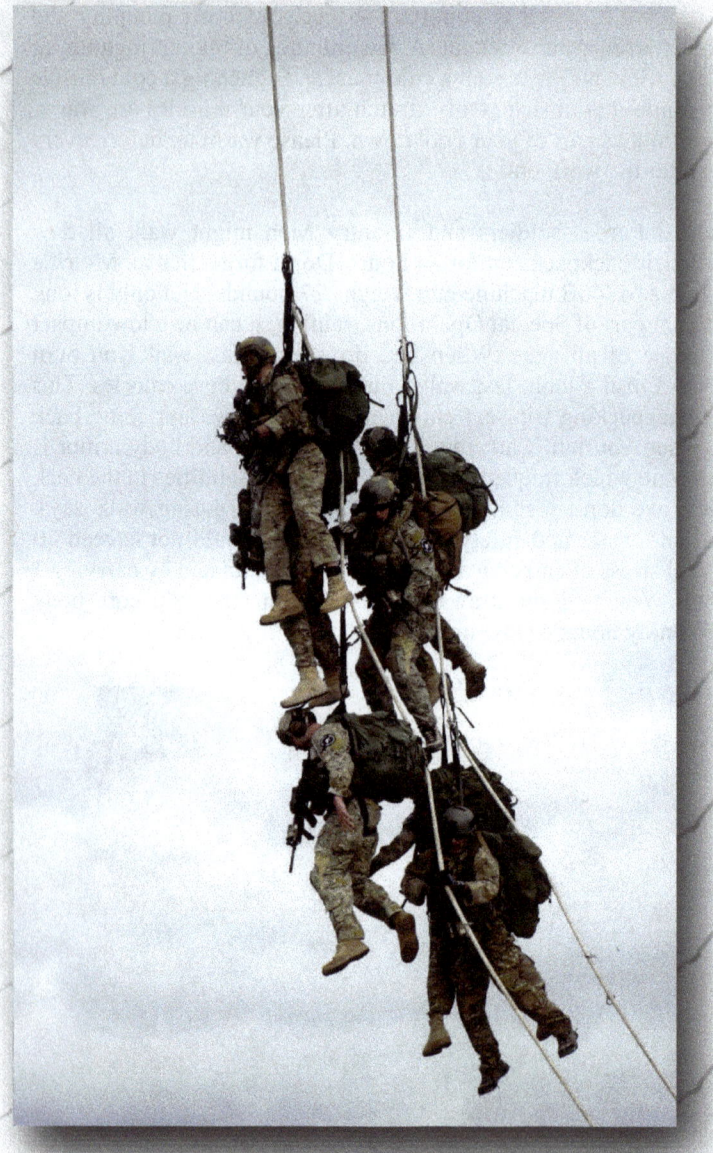

Safety First... Special Patrol Insertion & Exfiltration System (SPIES)
Public Domain U.S. Army photo by Spc. Steven Young

★ <u>Safety:</u> Special Operators have dangerous jobs. They rely on good safety habits to stay alive. They wear helmets, gloves, eye protection, use seatbelts in helicopters, and do rigorous SCUBA gear and Parachute inspections. Because we are not able to be there with you face to face, you need to be smart about protecting yourself.

<u>Seek medical approval prior to exercising.</u>

If you are a beginner, work up to doing the exercise with full body weight. Wear safety gear. Maintain situational awareness. Swim where there is a lifeguard present. Be safe. Life is a Special Operation.

SPECIAL OPERATIONS FITNESS

Week 0 Fitness Test

Week: 1
Day 1: United States
Day 2: Self Defense 1
Day 3: Canada
Weekend: Walk (2 hrs)

Week: 2
Day 1: Mexico
Day 2: Self Defense 2
Day 3: Guatemala
Weekend: Bike 1 "Tour de Neighborhood"

Week: 3
Day 1: Belize
Day 2: Self Defense 3
Day 3: Honduras
Weekend: Walk (3 hrs)

Week: 4
Day 1: El Salvador
Day 2: Self Defense 4
Day 3: Nicaragua
Weekend: Swim 1 "Tsunami"

Week: 5
Day 1: Costa Rica
Day 2: Self Defense 5
Day 3: Panama
Weekend: Walk (4 hrs)

Week: 6 "1000 Week"
Day 1: 200 Push Ups
Day 2: 200 Push Ups
Day 3: 200 Push Ups
Day 4: 200 Push Ups
Day 5: 200 Push Ups
Weekend: Cross Train 1

Week: 7
Day 1: United States
Day 2: Self Defense 6
Day 3: Canada
Weekend: Walk (5 hrs)

Week: 8
Day 1: Mexico
Day 2: Self Defense 2
Day 3: Guatemala
Weekend: Bike 2 "Seatless in Seattle"

Week: 9
Day 1: Belize
Day 2: Self Defense 4
Day 3: Honduras
Weekend: Walk (6 hrs)

Week: 10 "1000 Week"
Day 1: 200 Push Ups
Day 2: 200 Push Ups
Day 3: 200 Push Ups
Day 4: 200 Push Ups
Day 5: 200 Push Ups
Weekend: Swim 2 "Flash Flood"

Week: 11
Day 1: El Salvador
Day 2: Self Defense 6
Day 3: Nicaragua
Weekend: Walk (7 hrs)

Week: 12
Day 1: Costa Rica
Day 2: Self Defense 6
Day 3: Panama
Weekend: Cross Train 2

Life is a Special Operation. Are you Training for it?

Week 13 Fitness Test

SPECIAL OPERATIONS FITNESS

SPECIAL OPERATIONS FITNESS WORK OUTS

Fitness Test

- ★ Concept: This Fitness Test is conducted during "0 Week," before beginning Special Operations Fitness, and will measure your current state of physical fitness. At the end of 12 weeks you will take the identical test and will show exceptional physical fitness improvement. Please accurately record your results so you can more thoroughly see your improvement. We recommend taking before and after pictures. This will help motivate you. Feel free to post your results on our website (but remember, we only post photos of fully dressed Special Operations Fitness team members. "Mandex" is unauthorized). Congratulations in advance.
- ★ Duration: The Fitness Test should take no longer that 45 minutes. Take a few minutes to set up your testing facility and measure out your 25 meter Shuttle Run and 800 meter Sprint. Take the test in any order you want. Do not rest more than 5 minutes between events. Warm up before officially beginning the fitness test. Stretch immediately after finishing the fitness test.
- ★ Equipment Needed: Pull Up bar, blood pressure machine, stop watch.
- ★ Checklist / Record the following data:
    - Date with Before Picture
    - Body Weight, Body Fat Percentage, Calculated Weight of your Body Fat
    - Waste Size
    - Resting Heart Rate in Beats Per Minute
    - Blood Pressure (Measure before the fitness test but after sitting upright for 1 minute with arms and legs uncrossed)
    - # <u>Pull Ups</u> you can do with perfect form before dropping from the bar
    - # <u>Push Ups</u> you can do with perfect form before stopping or dropping to your knees
    - 800 meter Sprint time
    - 4x25 meter Shuttle Run time… Measure out 25m and mark it. Sprint from the start line to the 25m line, touch it. Sprint back to the start line, touch it. Sprint back to the 25m line, touch it. Sprint through the finish line. (100m total)
    - Time it takes to read the entire "Table of Contents" of this Special Operations Fitness 1.0 document out loud and up-side down

LIFE IS A SPECIAL OPERATION.COM

United States

★ Concept: At full intensity (but with control so you don't injure yourself) do the following circuit as many times as you can in 20 minutes. No rest between exercises.
  - 10 Pushups
  - 10 Dumbbell Bicep Curls
  - 10 Dumbbell Triceps Extensions
  - 10 Dumbbell Military Press
  - 10 Dumbbell Shoulder Shrugs
  - 20 Punching Sit-ups
★ Equipment Needed: A dumbbell which you can use for all exercises.
★ Note: Warm up before officially beginning the workout. Stretch immediately after finishing the workout. Do perfect form exercises to reduce the chance of injuries.
★ Beginners: Do "Beginner Variation" Push Ups from knees or against something evaluated. Always have good form and a full range of motion.
★ Experts: Do all exercises while balancing on one foot. This will help build support muscles and increase balance and agility.

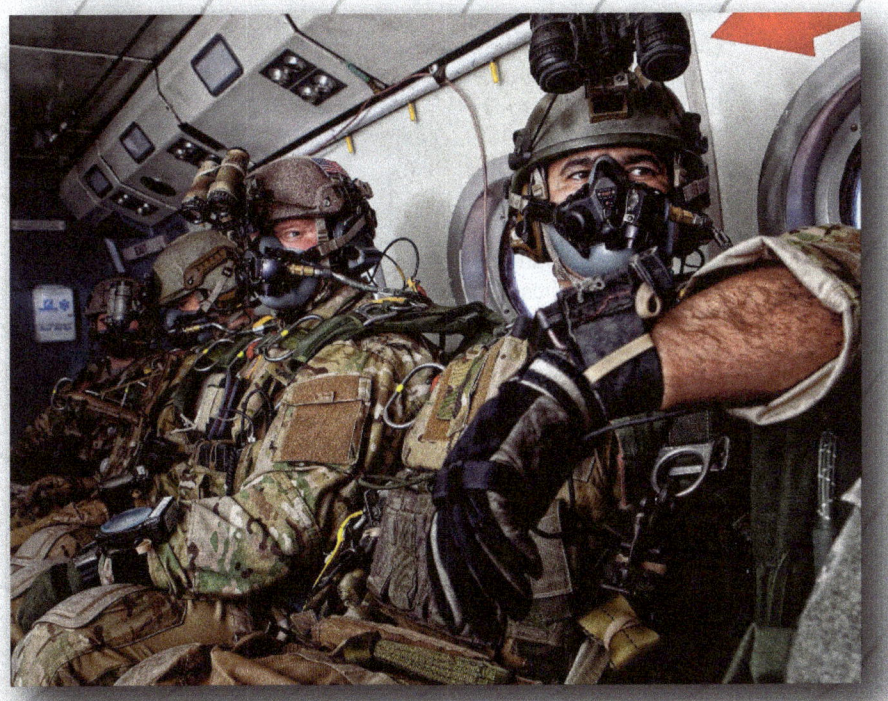

Before a High Altitude Low Opening (HALO) Parachute Infiltration Mission
Public Domain / U.S. Army John F. Kennedy Special Warfare Center

SPECIAL OPERATIONS FITNESS

[Canada](#)

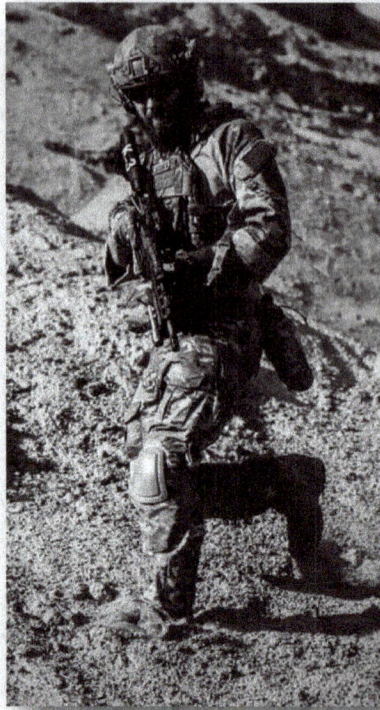

- ★ Concept: At full intensity (but with control so you don't injure yourself) do the following circuit. No rest between exercises.
    - 1 Pull Up, 10 Dumbbell Plank Rows, 10 Sit Ups to Hip Ups, 10 Dumbbell Overhead Snatches
    - 2 Pull Ups, 10 Dumbbell Plank Rows, 10 Sit Ups to Hip Ups, 10 Dumbbell Overhead Snatches
    - 3 Pull Ups, 10 Dumbbell Plank Rows, 10 Sit Ups to Hip Ups, 10 Dumbbell Overhead Snatches
    - 4 Pull Ups, 10 Dumbbell Plank Rows, 10 Sit Ups to Hip Ups, 10 Dumbbell Overhead Snatches
    - 5 Pull Ups, 10 Dumbbell Plank Rows, 10 Sit Ups to Hip Ups, 10 Dumbbell Overhead Snatches
    - 5 Pull Ups, 10 Dumbbell Plank Rows, 10 Sit Ups to Hip Ups, 10 Dumbbell Overhead Snatches
    - 4 Pull Ups, 10 Dumbbell Plank Rows, 10 Sit Ups to Hip Ups, 10 Dumbbell Overhead Snatches
    - 3 Pull Ups, 10 Dumbbell Plank Rows, 10 Sit Ups to Hip Ups, 10 Dumbbell Overhead Snatches
    - 2 Pull Ups, 10 Dumbbell Plank Rows, 10 Sit Ups to Hip Ups, 10 Dumbbell Overhead Snatches
    - 1 Pull Up, 10 Dumbbell Plank Rows, 10 Sit Ups to Hip Ups, 10 Dumbbell Overhead Snatches
- ★ Equipment Needed: Pull Up bar. A dumbbell which you can use for both exercises.
- ★ Note: Warm up before officially beginning the workout. Stretch immediately after finishing the workout. Do perfect form exercises to reduce the chance of injuries.
- ★ Beginners: Do "Beginner Variation" Pull Ups if you need to.
- ★ Experts: Do "Expert Variation" Pull Ups.

Special Forces Soldier

LIFE IS A SPECIAL OPERATION.COM

Mexico

- ★ Concept: At full intensity (but with control so you don't injure yourself) do the following circuit as many times as you can in 20 minutes. No rest between exercises.
    - o 10 Blast Off Push Ups
    - o 10 Break Dancers
    - o 10 Box Jumps
    - o 10 Dumbbell Snatches
    - o 10 Low Bar Pull Ups (feet further away from the bar)
    - o 10 Low Bar Pull Ups (feet closer to the bar)

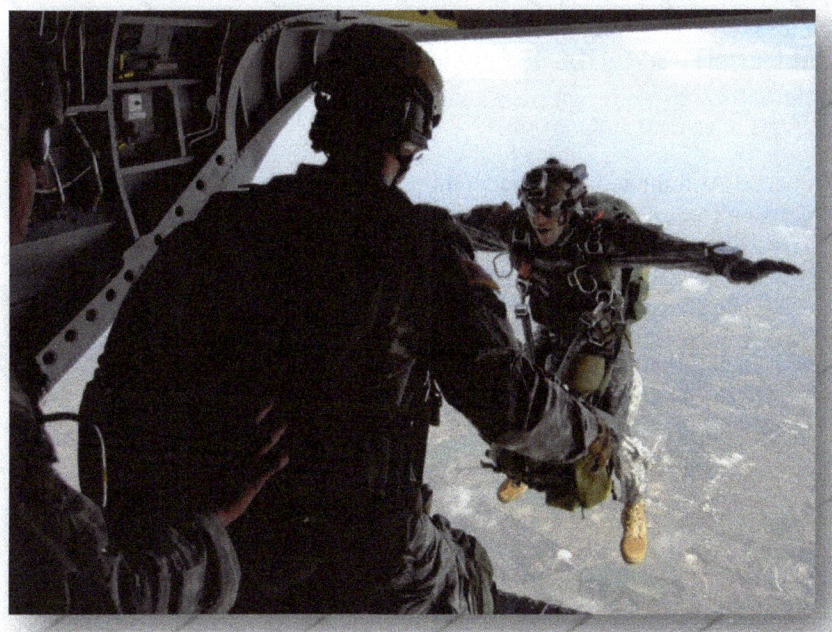

High Altitude Low Opening (HALO)
Parachute Infiltration Mission

- ★ Equipment Needed: Low Pull Up bar. A dumbbell for Snatches. A Box for Box Jumps.
- ★ Note: Warm up before officially beginning the workout. Stretch immediately after finishing the workout. Do perfect form exercises to reduce the chance of injuries.
- ★ Beginners: Do "Beginner Variations" for Push Ups once you can't do any more Blast Off Push Ups.
- ★ Experts: Do Low Bar Pull Ups while balancing on one foot. This will help build support muscles and increase balance and agility.

SPECIAL OPERATIONS FITNESS

Guatemala

- ★ Concept: At full intensity (but with control so you don't injure yourself) do the following circuit as many times as you can in 20 minutes. No rest between exercises.
    - 10 Side Jumps
    - 10 Man Makers
    - 10 Bent Over Rows (Dumbbells parallel with body)
    - 10 Bent Over Rows (Dumbbells perpendicular with body)
    - 20 Flutter Kicks
    - 10 Sit Ups to Hip Ups
- ★ Equipment Needed: Dumbbells.
- ★ Note: Warm up before officially beginning the workout. Stretch immediately after finishing the workout. Do perfect form exercises to reduce the chance of injuries.

Belize

- ★ Concept: At full intensity conduct the following track / sprint workout.
    - Sprint 100m, rest 1 minute
    - Sprint 100m, rest 1 minute
    - Sprint 200m, rest 1 minutes
    - Sprint 200m, rest 1 minute
    - Sprint 400m, rest 2 minute
    - Sprint 400m, rest 2 minute
    - Sprint 800m, rest 2 minute
    - Sprint 800m, rest 2 minute
    - Sprint 400m, rest 1 minute
    - Sprint 200m, rest 1 minute
    - Sprint 100m

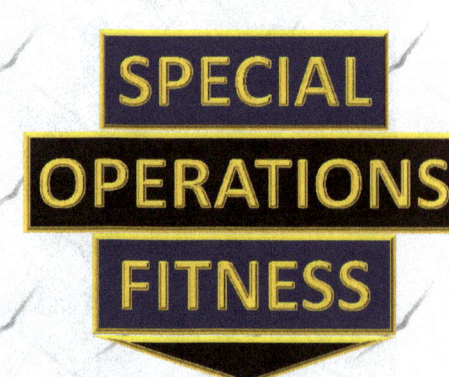

- ★ Equipment Needed: 400m running track. Or measure out a flat running surface with 100, 200, 400 & 800 meter marks.
- ★ Note: Warm up before officially beginning the workout. Stretch immediately after finishing the workout. Practice perfect running technique and give 100% effort.

El Salvador

- ★ Concept: At full intensity (but with control so you don't injure yourself) do the following circuit as many times as you can in 20 minutes. No rest between exercises.

    - o 10 Man Makers
    - o 10 Dumbbell Snatches
    - o 10 Low Bar Pull Ups (feet far out)
    - o 10 Low Bar Pull Ups (feet closer)

- ★ Equipment Needed: Low Pull Up bar. A dumbbell for Man Makers and Snatches.
- ★ Note: Warm up before officially beginning the workout. Stretch immediately after finishing the workout. Do perfect form exercises to reduce the chance of injuries.
- ★ Beginners: Do "Beginner Variations" for Push Ups once you can't do anymore.
- ★ Experts: Do Low Bar Pull Ups while balancing on one foot. This will help build support muscles and increase balance and agility.

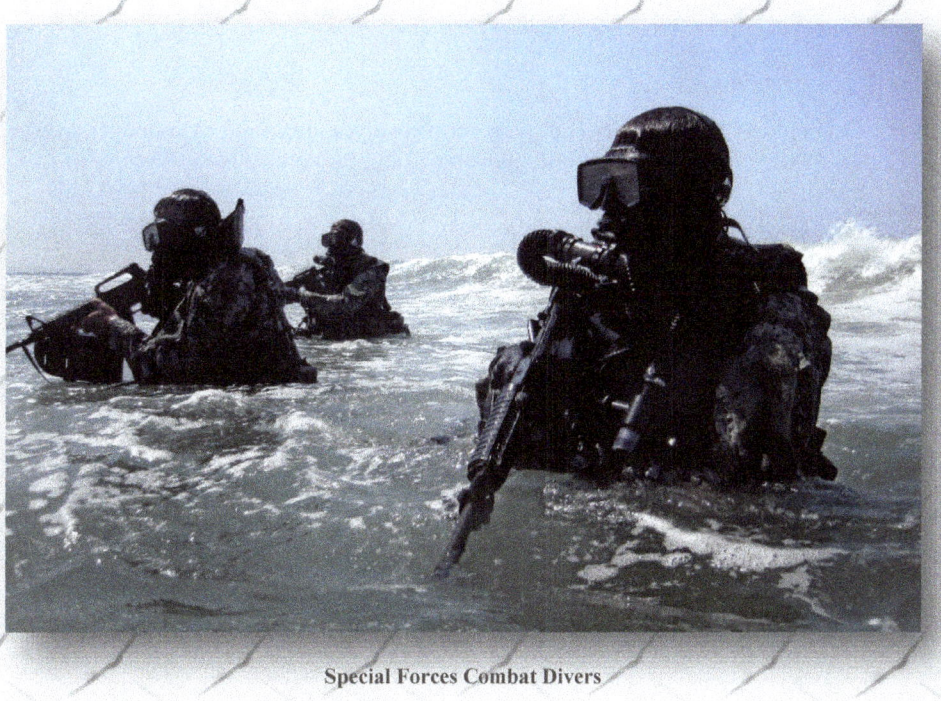

Special Forces Combat Divers

SPECIAL OPERATIONS FITNESS

Honduras

★ Concept: Today's workout requires precision. Exercise perfect form to prevent injury. Use a lighter dumbbell and do not rush. Do the following circuit as many times as you can in 20 minutes. No rest between exercises.
- 1 minute High Knees
- 10 Ins and Outs
- 10 Ups and Downs
- 10 Twisters
- 10 Plank Tricep Extensions
- 10 Break Dancers
- 10 Bent Over Rows (Dumbbells parallel with body)
- 10 Bent Over Rows (Dumbbells perpendicular with body)

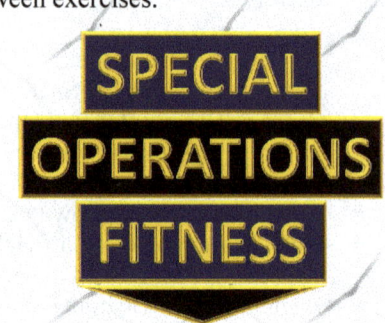

★ Equipment Needed: Dumbbells for rotational exercises.
★ Note: Warm up before officially beginning the workout. Stretch immediately after finishing the workout. Do perfect form exercises to reduce the chance of injuries.

Nicaragua

★ Concept: At full intensity (but with control so you don't injure yourself) do the following circuit as many times as you can in 20 minutes. No rest between exercises.
- 10 Blast Off Push Ups
- 10 Box Jumps
- 10 Star Jumps
- 1 Minute High Knees
- 10 Side Jumpers
- 25 meter Walking Lunge
- 10 Hip Ups
- 25 meter Sprint

★ Equipment Needed: Box.
★ Note: Warm up before officially beginning the workout. Stretch immediately after finishing the workout. Do perfect form exercises to reduce the chance of injuries.
★ Beginners: Do "Beginner Variations" for Push Ups once you can't do any more Blast Off Push Ups.

LIFE IS A SPECIAL OPERATION.COM

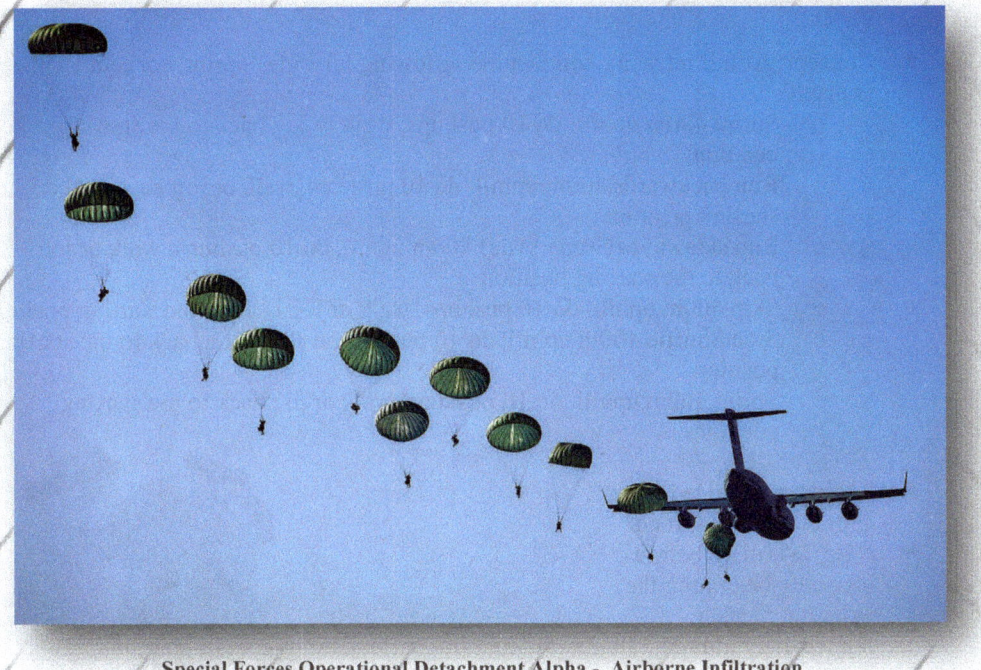

Special Forces Operational Detachment Alpha - Airborne Infiltration

Costa Rica

★ Concept: At full intensity (but with control so you don't injure yourself) do 20 minutes of Traveling Man Makers with very light Dumbbells. Record how far you travel.
★ Equipment Needed: 5 or 10 pound Dummbells. A safe road or track.
★ Note: Warm up before officially beginning the workout. Stretch immediately after finishing the workout. Do perfect form exercises to reduce the chance of injuries.

SPECIAL OPERATIONS FITNESS

Panama

- ★ Concept: At full intensity conduct the following hill side / sprint workout. Time yourself.
    - Sprint 400m uphill, do 10 pushups, walk or jog back to the starting position
    - Run backwards 400m uphill, do 10 pushups, walk or jog back to the starting position
    - Run sideways (Grape Vine) 400m uphill, do 10 pushups, walk or jog back to the starting position
    - Skip 400m uphill, do 10 pushups, walk or jog back to the starting position
    - Side Shuffle 400m uphill, do 10 pushups, walk or jog back to the starting position
    - Sprint 400m uphill, do 10 pushups, walk or jog back to the starting position

- ★ Equipment Needed: 400m long hill or road.
- ★ Note: Warm up before officially beginning the workout. Stretch immediately after finishing the workout. When running sideways or doing the side shuffling, alternate sides every 100 meters. Do pushups facing uphill.
- ★ Beginners: Take it easy on your side-run and side-shuffle speeds if you feel unstable. Do Pushups from knees or against something evaluated.
- ★ Experts: Do "expert variations" for your pushups.

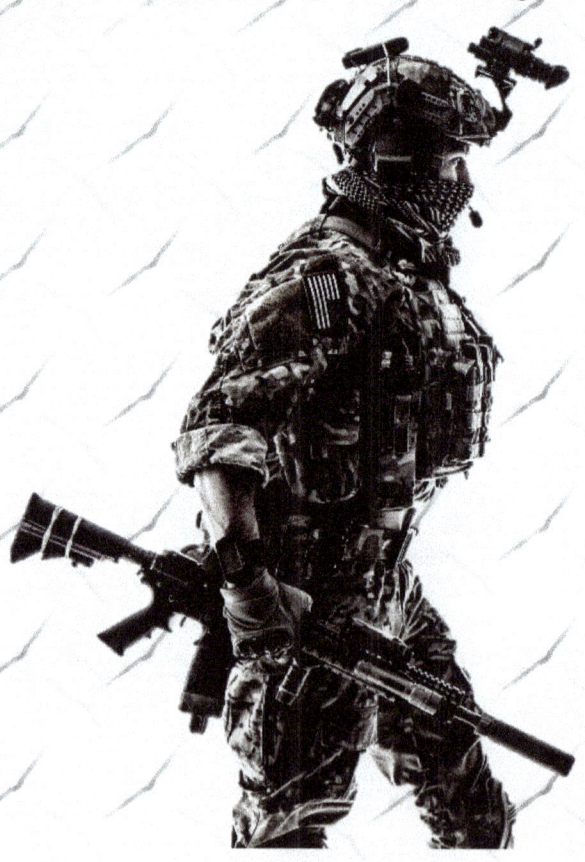

LIFE IS A SPECIAL OPERATION.COM

Self Defense 1

- ★ Concept: At full intensity (but with control so you don't injure yourself) do the following circuit five times.
    - o 50 left hand jabs
    - o 50 right hand jabs
    - o 50 left hand punches
    - o 50 right hand punches
    - o 50 hooks/ upper cuts (1 left then 1 right) 100 total
    - o 2 minutes rest
- ★ Equipment Needed: Hand wraps, bag gloves, heavy bag.
- ★ Note: Warm up before officially beginning the workout. Stretch immediately after finishing the workout. Do perfect form strikes. Never do a sloppy strike. If you get tired, then slow down. Build muscle memory via perfect technique.

Self Defense 2

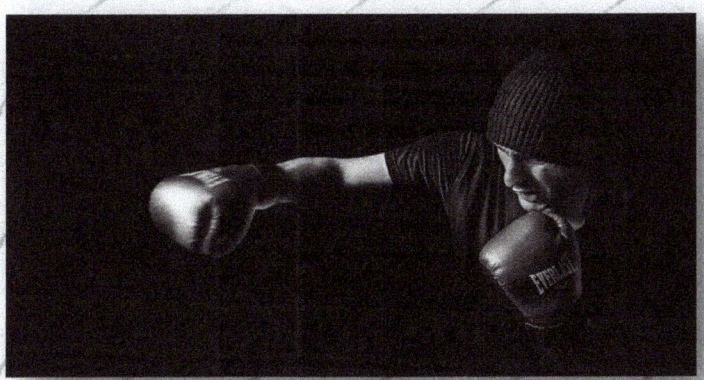

The Jab has broken more noses than any other Punch or Kick

- ★ Concept: At full intensity (but with control so you don't injure yourself) do the following circuit 5 times:
    - o 50 repetitions of 2 left hand jabs followed by 1 right hand punch
    - o 50 repetitions of 2 right hand jabs followed by 1 left hand punch
    - o 50 repetitions of 2 left hand jabs followed by 1 right hand punch, then a left hook
    - o 50 repetitions of 2 right hand jabs followed by 1 left hand punch, then a right hook
    - o 2 minutes rest
- ★ Equipment Needed: Hand wraps, bag gloves, heavy bag.
- ★ Note: Warm up before officially beginning the workout. Stretch immediately after finishing the workout. Do perfect form strikes. Never do a sloppy strike. If you get tired, then slow down. Build muscle memory via perfect technique.

SPECIAL OPERATIONS FITNESS

Self Defense 3

- ★ Concept: At full intensity (but with control so you don't injure yourself) spar with the heavy bag for three minutes then rest for two minutes. Use only punching techniques. Repeat six times.
- ★ Equipment Needed: Hand wraps, bag gloves, heavy bag.
- ★ Note: Warm up before officially beginning the workout. Stretch immediately after finishing the workout. Do perfect form strikes. Never do a sloppy strike. If you get tired, then slow down. Build muscle memory via perfect technique.

Self Defense 4

- ★ Concept: At full intensity (but with control so you don't injure yourself) do the following circuit five times.
    - 20 right rear leg front kicks
    - 20 left rear leg front kicks
    - 20 right front leg front kicks
    - 20 left front leg front kicks
    - 20 right rear leg round kicks
    - 20 left rear leg round kicks
    - 20 right front leg round kicks
    - 20 left front leg round kicks
    - 2 minutes rest
- ★ Equipment Needed: Heavy bag.
- ★ Note: Warm up before officially beginning the workout. Stretch immediately after finishing the workout. Keep your hands up to protect your face. Do perfect form kicks. Never do a sloppy kick. If you get tired, then slow down. Build muscle memory via perfect technique.

Self Defense 5

- ★ Concept: At full intensity (but with control so you don't injure yourself) spar with the heavy bag for three minutes then rest for 2 minutes. Use punches and kicks. Repeat 6 times.
- ★ Equipment Needed: Hand wraps, bag gloves, heavy bag.
- ★ Note: Warm up before officially beginning the workout. Stretch immediately after finishing the workout. Do perfect form punches and kicks. Never do a sloppy punch or kick. If you get tired, then slow down. Build muscle memory via perfect technique.

Self Defense 6

★ Concept: At full intensity - conduct the following six heavy bag circuits.
- Round 1:
  - 50 left hand jabs
  - 50 right hand jabs
  - 50 left hand punches
  - 50 right hand punches
  - 50 hooks or upper cuts (1 left then 1 right) 100 total
  - 2 minutes rest
- Round 2:
  - 20 right rear leg front kicks
  - 20 left rear leg front kicks
  - 20 right front leg front kicks
  - 20 left front leg front kicks
  - 20 right rear leg round kicks
  - 20 left rear leg round kicks
  - 20 right front leg round kicks
  - 20 left front leg round kicks
  - 2 minutes rest

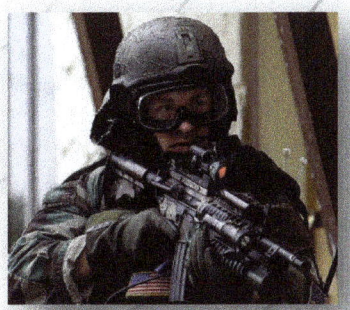

A Special Forces Soldier prepares to breach an entryway while training in close quarters battle tactics at Fort Bragg, N.C. (U.S. Army Special Operations Command photo)

- Round 3:
  - 50 left hand jabs
  - 50 right hand jabs
  - 50 left hand punches
  - 50 right hand punches
  - 50 hooks (1 left then 1 right) 100 total
  - 2 minutes rest
- Round 4:
  - 20 right rear leg front kicks
  - 20 left rear leg front kicks
  - 20 right front leg front kicks
  - 20 left front leg front kicks
  - 20 right rear leg round kicks
  - 20 left rear leg round kicks
  - 20 right front leg round kicks
  - 20 left front leg round kicks
  - 2 minutes rest
- Round 5: Three minute spar with heavy bag using kicks and punches. Rest two minutes.
- Round 6: Three minute spar with heavy bag using kicks and punches.

SPECIAL OPERATIONS FITNESS

- ★ Equipment Needed: Hand wraps, bag gloves, heavy bag
- ★ Note: Warm up before officially beginning the workout. Stretch immediately after finishing the workout. Do perfect form punches and kicks. Never do a sloppy punch or kick. If you get tired, then slow down. Build muscle memory via perfect technique.

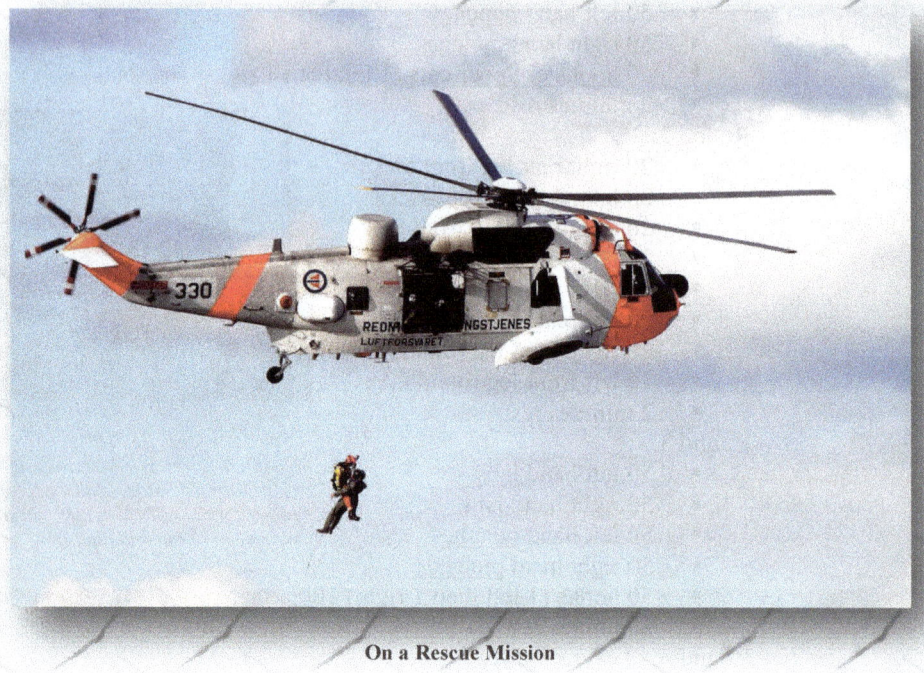

On a Rescue Mission

Bike 1 "Tour De Neighborhood"

- ★ Concept: Go for a bicycle ride outside for 35 minutes. The first five minutes should be a warm up. The next 30 minutes are bicycle sprint circuits. During this time you must sprint (100% effort) on the bicycle for 3 minutes then return to a quick speed (75%) for 2 minutes. Repeat this circuit 6 times.
- ★ Equipment Needed: A bicycle and safety gear.
- ★ Note: Warm up before officially beginning the workout. Stretch immediately after finishing the workout.

LIFE IS A SPECIAL OPERATION.COM

Bike 2 "Seatless in Seattle"

* Concept: Take off your seat (and seat post) or lower your seat all the way. Don't use it during this workout. Go for a bicycle ride outside for 35 minutes. The first five minutes should be a warm up. The next 30 minutes are bicycle sprint circuits. During this time you must sprint (100% effort) on the bicycle for 3 minutes then return to a quick speed (75%) for 2 minutes. Repeat this circuit 6 times.
* Equipment Needed: A bicycle and safety gear.
* Note: Warm up before officially beginning the workout. Stretch immediately after finishing the workout.

Swim 1 "Tsunami"

* Concept: Jump into the pool and swim to the other side underwater. Come up when you need more air. Do this as many times as you need to in order to get to the other side. Once you reach the other side, get out of the pool and do 10 perfect form pushups. Get back into the pool and swim free style (aka the crawl) back to the other side of the pool. Once you reach the other side, get out of the pool and to 10 perfect form flutter kicks. Repeat. Keep up this circuit for 20 minutes. Give 100%.

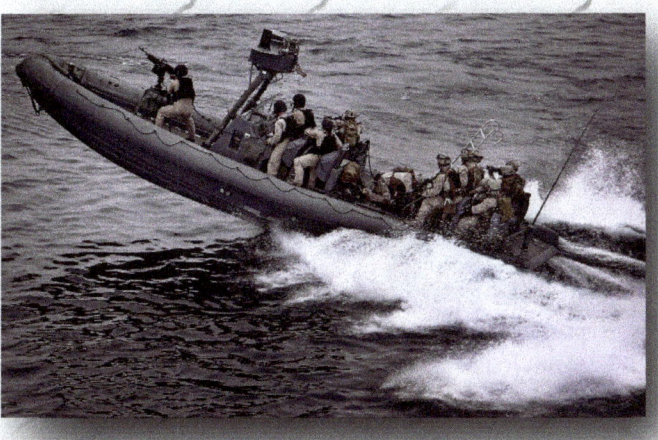

Special Warfare Combatant-Craft Crewmen (SWCC)

* Equipment Needed: 25 meter swimming pool, pants and t-shirt, swim goggles if you prefer.
* Note: Wear pants and a t-shirt for this workout. Warm up before officially beginning the workout. Stretch immediately after finishing the workout. Ensure that the necessary lifeguards are there.
* Weak or Non-Swimmers: Don't worry. There is no shame in not being a good swimmer. But please learn to swim as this is an important life skill.
    o Option 1 is to do the workout but don't swim underwater. Simply stay on the surface and do the best that you can.
    o Option 2 is to use the side of the pool and the lane lines to pull yourself from one side of the pool to the other (remember, keep up the intensity).
    o Option 3 is to do 50 meter sprints instead of the swim. Alternate 10 pushups and 10 flutter kicks at each side.

SPECIAL OPERATIONS FITNESS

Swim 2 "Flash Flood"

★ Concept: Take two old t-shirts and put one in each hand. Jump into the pool and swim free style (aka the crawl) to the other side. Once you reach the other side, get out of the pool and do 10 perfect form pushups. Get back into the pool and swim back to the other side of the pool. Once you reach the other side, get out of the pool and to 10 perfect form flutter kicks. Repeat. Keep up this circuit for 20 minutes. Give 100%.

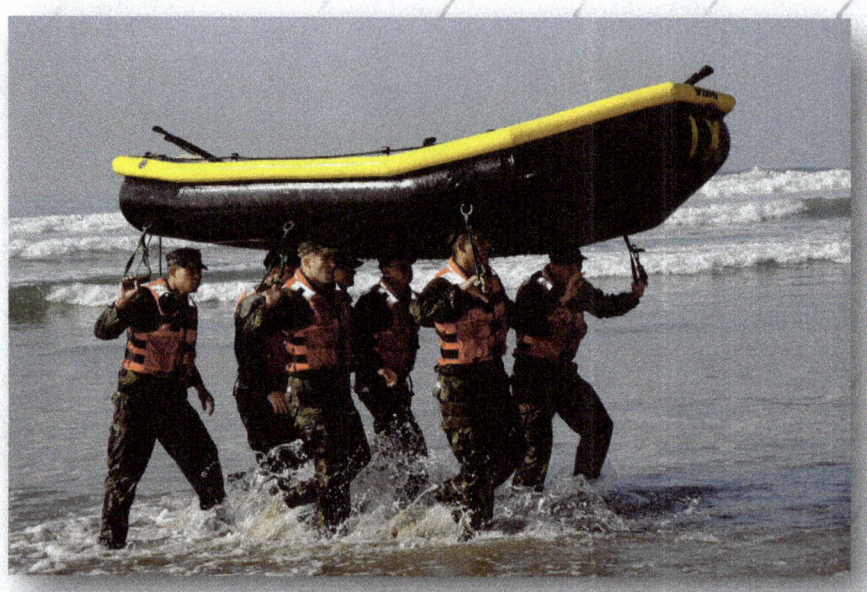

Navy Seal Training

★ Equipment Needed: 2 old t-shirts, 25 meter swimming pool, pants and t-shirt, goggles if you prefer.
★ Note: Wear pants and a t-shirt for this workout. Warm up before officially beginning the workout. Stretch immediately after finishing the workout. Ensure that the necessary lifeguards are there.
★ Weak or Non-Swimmers: Don't worry. There is no shame in not being a good swimmer. But please learn to swim as this is an important life skill.
  o Option 1 is to do the workout but don't hold the t-shirts in each hand.
  o Option 2 is to use the side of the pool and the lane lines to pull yourself from one side of the pool to the other (remember, keep up the intensity).
  o Option 3 is to do 50 meter sprints instead of the swim. Alternate 10 pushups and 10 flutter kicks at each side.

LIFE IS A SPECIAL OPERATION.COM

"1000 Week"

★ Concept: Do 200 perfect form pushups every day for 5 days. This makes 1000 pushups in a week. Experts should do 4 sets of 50 perfect form pushups each day. Beginners can do 20 sets of 10 perfect form pushups each day. If you can't do 10 regular pushups then do them from your knees or against something elevated. Spread the pushups throughout the day. For example, a moderately fit person does 10 sets of 20 perfect form pushups, one set every hour.

★ Note: Warm up before each set of pushups. You will be sore.

Cross Train 1 & 2

★ Concept: Do 30 minutes of 100% effort, high intensity cross training. We recommend not running or sprinting to give your knees a rest. Perhaps you can bike, row, kayak, swim, rock climb, etc. Enjoy, but give it 100% effort.

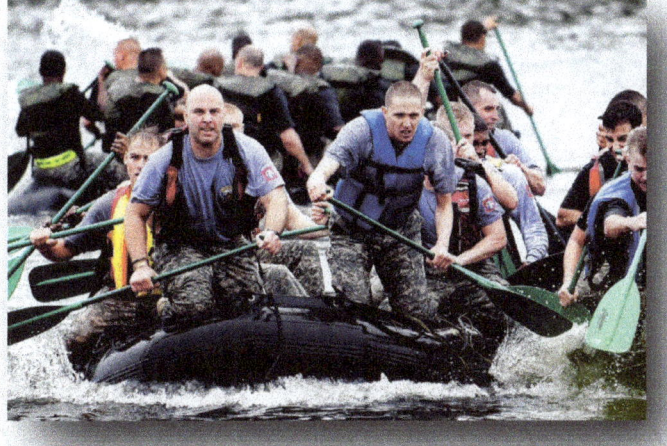

Soldiers doing a Boat Work Out

★ Note: Warm up before officially beginning the workout. Stretch immediately after finishing the workout.

2 or 3 Hour Walks

★ Concept: At a pace of 4 miles per hour or faster walk nonstop for 2 or 3 hours straight. Keep a 3-5 pound dumbbell in your hands and alternate carrying the dumbbell with equal time in each hand.

★ Equipment Needed: A 3-5 pound dumbbell. An iPod or MP3 player is optional.

★ Note: Warm up before officially beginning the workout. Stretch immediately after finishing the workout. Walk, don't run.

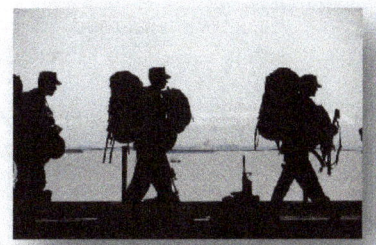

Carrying Everything They Have

Walk to the mall, through the woods, into town, home from work, etc. Use your

SPECIAL OPERATIONS FITNESS

imagination. Don't get lost. Bring appropriate safety gear if going through the forest or reflective gear if walking at night. If you do bring an iPod or MP3 then listen to a book on tape, the bible, a motivational speaker, etc. Don't listen to music but listen to something which makes you smarter. Maintain situational awareness if using ear phones so you aren't hit by a car, bike, or bear. Have good walking form with head up, back straight. No slouching.

- ★ Experts: Bring a small backpack with food, water, safety gear. Do not exceed 30 pounds.

4, 5, 6 or 7 Hour Walks

- ★ Concept: At a pace of about 4 miles per hour, walk nonstop for 4, 5, 6, or 7 hours straight. Keep a 3-5 pound dumbbell in your hands and alternate carrying the dumbbell with equal time in each hand.
- ★ Equipment Needed: A 3-5 pound dumbbell. An iPod or MP3 player is optional.
- ★ Note: Warm up before officially beginning the workout. Stretch immediately after finishing the workout. Walk, don't run. Walk to the mall, through the woods, into town, home from work, etc. Use your imagination. Don't get lost. Bring appropriate safety gear if going through the forest or reflective gear if walking at night. If you do bring an iPod or MP3 then listen to a book on tape, the bible, a motivational speaker, etc. Don't listen to music but listen to something which makes you smarter. Maintain situational awareness if using ear phones so you aren't hit by a car, bike, or bear. Have good walking form with head up, back straight. No slouching.
- ★ Beginners: Bring a small backpack with food, water, safety gear. Don't overload yourself.
- ★ Experts: Bring a small backpack with food, water, safety gear. Do not exceed 30 pounds.

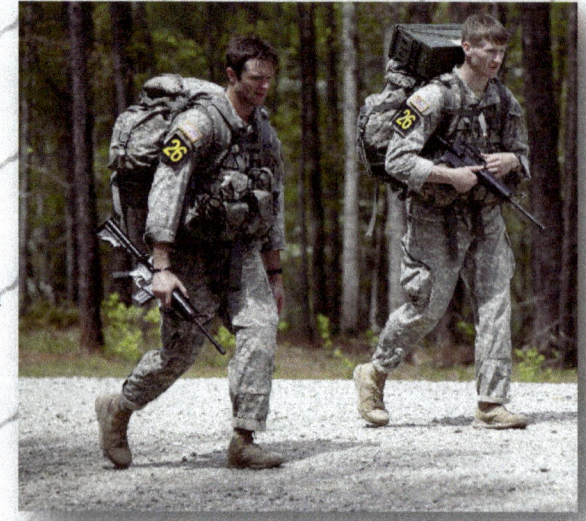

... Literally Walking All Day Long
Best Ranger Competition
Public Domain Photo by Sgt. Austin Berner

LIFE IS A SPECIAL OPERATION.COM

5 ESSENTIAL TRAINING TIPS TO PREPARE FOR SPECIAL FORCES OR DELTA FORCE SELECTION (TRY OUTS)

I have been asked thousands of times how to prepare for Special Forces Selection (Try Outs). Below you will find my pragmatic recommendations. Even if you are not going to Selection, learning how to toughen your feet, shoulders, and back will help make you a faster hiker, a better backpacker, and a stronger person.

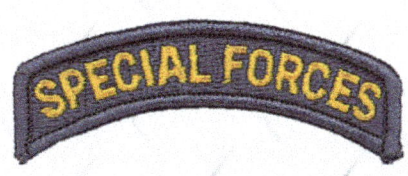

1) Walk A Lot: At Selection, you will be patrolling where you literally walk all day long. You will conduct Land Navigation courses where you literally walk all day long. It is insufficient to go for a 12 mile Ruck March every weekend to train for "Selection." A 12 mile Ruck March only takes three hours. Walking for three hours is not a way to train for a competition where you will walk for 24 hours. When I say "walk a lot" I mean every weekend try to walk 8-12 hours a day. This will condition your body to being on your feet and constantly moving.

2) Wear your Back Pack a lot. The same logic from above applies. Wearing a 45 pound back pack during a three hour Ruck March is not a good way to train for an competition where you will wear your Ruck Sack 24 hours straight. Get your shoulders and back accustomed to wearing your military issued Ruck Sack. When it is "weird" to be seen with a military Ruck Sack, wear a discrete civilian style back pack. Wear it everywhere. Wear it to the mall or grocery shopping. Hike in it. Carry it to and from your Office.

3) Harden Your Feet: If you get blisters at Selection you are done. Bloody feet have made hundreds of strong men quit before reaching the finish line. So harden your feet before you go. Walk with-out socks once a week. Poor water into your boots every few Ruck Marches to simulate walking in the rain. Alternate boots. Never train by walking on a road. Walking on a road lets you take consistent steps. At Selection, you will be walking cross country, up, down, and sideways across hills and mountains. This places a lot of friction on your feet. Only train while walking cross country or on the rough shoulder, parallel to a road.

4) Have 2 Pairs of Good Boots: Make sure you have at least two pairs of good boots which are broken in and ready for six weeks of hard abuse. Breaking in new boots while at Selection is not advisable. Arriving with old boots which fall apart the last week of Selection is also not advisable. Plan ahead. Better to spend $125 two months before Selection than to be in a position where your old boots fail you.

SPECIAL OPERATIONS FITNESS

5) Orienteering: Because Orienteering / Land Navigation is an important part of the Selection process, I recommend that you become an expert at navigating with a map and compass before you go to selection.

THE 6TH ESSENTIAL TRAINING TIPS TO PREPARE FOR RANGER SCHOOL

Getting prepared for Ranger School is very similar to preparing for "Selection." The above listed 5 Training Tips also apply. But when preparing for Ranger School, I have an unconventional, but absolutely brilliant 6th Training Tip.

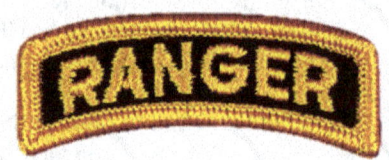

6) Get as fat as you can, but still be able to run 5 miles in 40 minutes while tired:

The worse part of Ranger School is 72 days of being cold, wet, hungry, and sleep deprived. Everyone loses weight at Ranger School and those who graduate are "lean and mean." I have weighed over 220 pounds while on Active Duty Special Forces. But I graduated from Ranger School at 160 pounds. No matter what, Ranger School is miserable. But the best way to make Ranger School less miserable is to show up with a lot of body fat. You are going to lose that fat for sure. But having that fat reserve helps keep you a little warmer and gives you a small energy reserve.

The single event which Ranger Students dread the most is the 5 mile run, which has a 40 minute time requirement. By itself, 5 miles in 40 minutes is easy. What makes this event so hard is that you are already starved and sleep deprived when you have to do your 5 mile run at 3 o'clock in the morning. So get as fat as you can before going to ranger school, but still be able to run 5 miles in 40 minutes while tired.

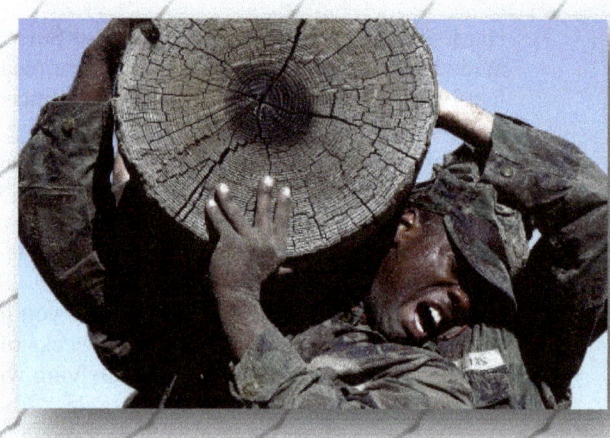

Log P.T. (Physical Training)

LIFE IS A SPECIAL OPERATION.COM

SPECIAL OPERATIONS FITNESS EXERCISES

We have created a video for you which demonstrates the exercises used during the Special Operations Fitness workouts. You must be online to watch.

1. Pull Ups
2. Low Bar Pull Ups
3. Push Ups
4. Blast Off Push Ups
5. Plank Rows
6. Plank Triceps Extensions
7. Break Dancers
8. Overhead Snatches
9. Box Jumps
10. Star Jumps
11. Side Jumpers
12. Walking Lunge
13. Hip Ups
14. Sit Ups to Hip Ups
15. Bicep Curl
16. Triceps Extension
17. Military Press
18. Shoulder Shrugs
19. Man Makers
20. Traveling Man Makers
21. Ins and Outs
22. Ups and Downs
23. Twisters
24. Bent Over Rows (Dumbbells parallel with body)
25. Bent Over Rows (Dumbbells perpendicular with body)
26. Flutter Kick
27. Punching Sit-ups
28. High Knees
29. 25 meter Shuttle Run
30. Backwards Run
31. Skip
32. Side Run (Grapevine)
33. Side Shuffle

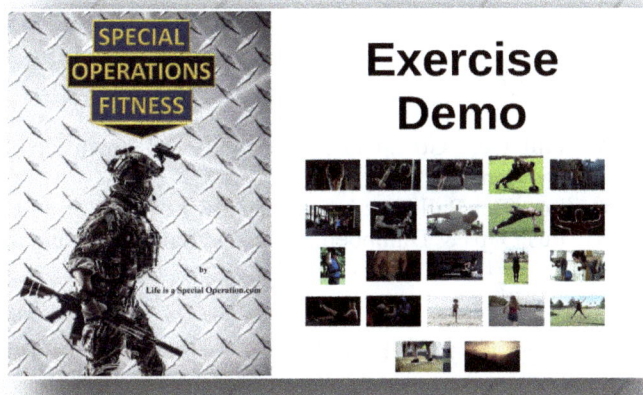

Special Operations Fitness Exercise Demonstrations
(YouTube)

SPECIAL OPERATIONS FITNESS

Beginner Variations

- ★ Pull Ups: (1) Strengthen your biceps and back muscles with Low Bar Pull Ups. No kipping or swinging. (2) Try doing "Negatives" where you jump to the up position then slowly let gravity pull you back down.
- ★ Low Bar Pull Ups: Use a higher Low Bar to make it easier on your biceps and back muscles. Build up to a normal level Low Bar.
- ★ Push Ups: Do pushups from your knees or against something elevated (a tree, rock, chair).

Expert Variations

- ★ Pull Ups: Go up fast (1 second) and down slowly (5 seconds). No kipping or swinging.
- ★ Low Bar Pull Ups: Use a very low Low Bar or do Low Bar Pull Ups with one arm.
- ★ Push Ups & Dumbbell Exercises: Balance on one foot while doing the exercise.

SPECIAL OPERATIONS FITNESS SELF DEFENSE TECHNIQUES

We have created a video for you which demonstrates all the Techniques used during the Special Operations Fitness Self Defense workouts. You must be online to watch.

1. Jab
2. Punch
3. Hook / Upper Cut
4. Front Leg Front Kick
5. Rear Led Front Kick
6. Front Leg Round Kick
7. Rear Leg Round Kick

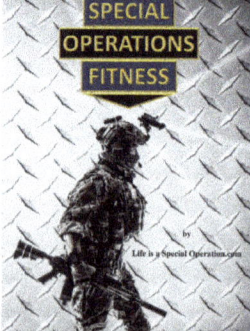
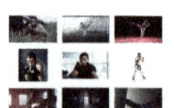

Special Operations Fitness Self Defense Technique Demonstrations (YouTube)

LIFE IS A SPECIAL OPERATION.COM

CONCLUSION

We have now given you an unconventional workout program which contains:

- ★ 12 weeks of dumbbell and body-weight boot-camp style workouts which use variations of 33 different exercises
- ★ 6 exhausting self-defense kick-boxing workouts
- ★ 2 lung crushing swim workouts
- ★ 2 unique biking workouts
- ★ 2 flexible cross training workouts
- ★ 6 hikes

Take a few minutes to plan ahead for your fitness test, and get yourself organized and prepared for your new challenge.

All it takes now is 12 weeks and the discipline to stick to the fitness plan.

Don't forget to let us know how Special Operations Fitness has changed your life.

We congratulate you in advanced.

Now....get to work!

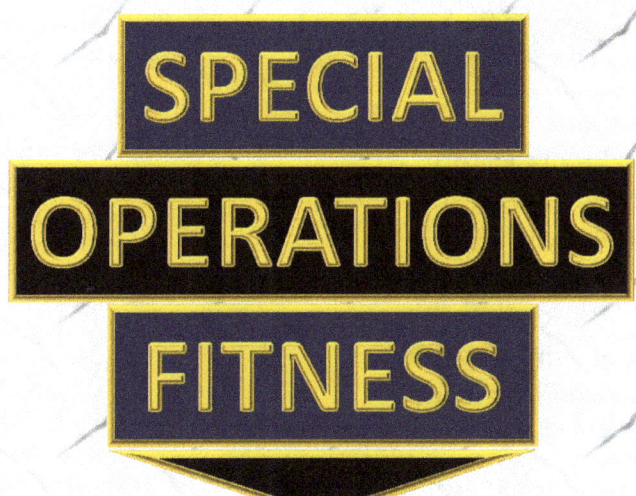

SPECIAL OPERATIONS FITNESS

SPECIAL OPERATIONS FITNESS

Weeks 1-6 Check List

- ☐ United States
- ☐ Canada
- ☐ Mexico
- ☐ Guatemala
- ☐ Belize
- ☐ Honduras
- ☐ El Salvador
- ☐ Nicaragua
- ☐ Costa Rica
- ☐ Panama
- ☐ Walk 2 hrs
- ☐ Walk 3 hrs
- ☐ Walk 4 hrs
- ☐ Bike 1 "Tour de Neighborhood"
- ☐ Swim 1 "Tsunami"
- ☐ 1000 Week
- ☐ Cross Train 1
- ☐ Self Defense 1
- ☐ Self Defense 2
- ☐ Self Defense 3
- ☐ Self Defense 4
- ☐ Self Defense 5

Week 0 Fitness Test

- ☐ Date:
- ☐ Before Picture
- ☐ Body Weight:
- ☐ Body Fat %:
- ☐ Weight of Body Fat:
- ☐ Waste Size:
- ☐ Resting Heart Rate:
- ☐ Blood Pressure:
- ☐ # Pull Ups:
- ☐ # Push Ups:
- ☐ 800m Sprint Time:
- ☐ 4x25m Shuttle Run Time:
- ☐ Upside Down Reading Time:

Weeks 7-12 Check List

- ☐ United States
- ☐ Canada
- ☐ Mexico
- ☐ Guatemala
- ☐ Belize
- ☐ Honduras
- ☐ El Salvador
- ☐ Nicaragua
- ☐ Costa Rica
- ☐ Panama
- ☐ Walk 5 hrs
- ☐ Walk 6 hrs
- ☐ Walk 7 hrs
- ☐ Bike 2 "Seatless in Seattle"
- ☐ Swim 2 "Flash Flood"
- ☐ 1000 Week
- ☐ Cross Train 2
- ☐ Self Defense 6
- ☐ Self Defense 2
- ☐ Self Defense 4
- ☐ Self Defense 6
- ☐ Self Defense 6

LIFE IS A SPECIAL OPERATION.COM

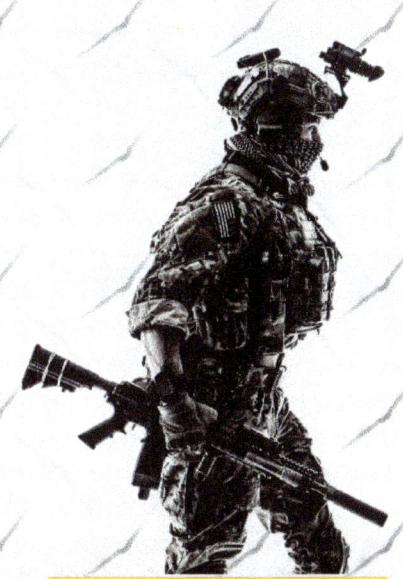

Week 13 Fitness Test

- ☐ Date:
- ☐ Before Picture
- ☐ Body Weight:
- ☐ Body Fat %:
- ☐ Weight of Body Fat:
- ☐ Waste Size:
- ☐ Resting Heart Rate:
- ☐ Blood Pressure:
- ☐ # Pull Ups:
- ☐ # Sit Ups:
- ☐ 800m Sprint Time:
- ☐ 4x25m Shuttle Run Time:
- ☐ Upside Down Reading Time:

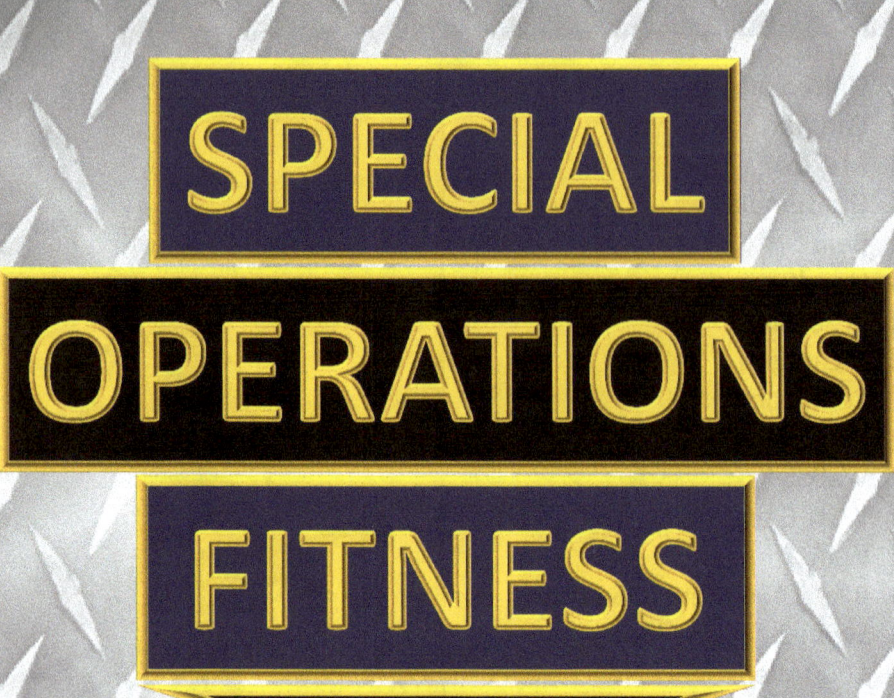

by
Life is a Special Operation.com

www.ingramcontent.com/pod-product-compliance
Lightning Source LLC
Chambersburg PA
CBHW070037040426
42333CB00040B/1712